The Ultimate Guide to Healthy Aging

A balanced approach to health and wellbeing

By Shiv Kumar

Disclaimer

The information provided in this book is intended for informational and educational purposes only. It is not a substitute for professional medical advice, diagnosis, or treatment.

PREFACE

You only live once. So, why not make the best of this life that you have got? Perhaps, majority of the people want to actually do this.

But there is a problem. The body gives up after a certain age. Sometimes, you are drained even mentally and emotionally. And then, all your dreams and aspirations just fade away with a lack of good health. Did you see the problem here?

But don't worry, this book is precisely here to help you in this regard. It will assist you to maintain, build, and improve your fitness as you age. I know it sounds difficult. In reality, it's not, if you make adequate efforts in the right direction.

Let me give you an analogy. Imagine you bought a new car. You used it for a year and you used it roughly on all terrains with no issues. But then slowly the wear and tear start to become evident. And since you did not service the car and also used it improperly, you may now have a real hard time behind the wheel.

But if you would have taken care of the car and serviced it properly, it would have definitely offered you a smooth ride for years.

Just like a car, your body is also a machine in a way. And it needs proper care and maintenance. Only when you service it properly, can it function smoothly. In this book, I will help you achieve maximum health and fitness in your life as you age. I know there will be problems and the solutions will not be instant. But gradually, you should definitely see progress. It is a process that takes time.

And the best thing is, the earlier you start working to build and maintain your health, the better it is for you. Because as they say, "prevention is better than cure," it will take way less effort and time now than in the future when your health may have deteriorated to a greater extent.

Sure, this era is very advanced. There are things like Biohacking, AI, Health Trackers, and a lot of other gadgets. And you may also be able to restore your health when you are a little older. But if you keep it for later, the amount of time and effort that it will take for the desired outcome will grow manifold.

The choice is yours! If you ask me, I will say there is no better time than 'today' to start working on your health.

Just to be transparent, I am not in my 50's or 60's, but I have been able to improve my fitness and health to a great extent with sustained efforts and god's grace, to be able to live a much healthful life now. My age is nearing 40 now. I can jog, run, swim, play, and work with more ease now compared to a few years earlier. This was made possible by following certain changes in my daily life. And this should apply to people of all age groups. Of course, there would be some custom changes based on which you may have to practice things that would work best for you. But overall, this book should work for all the ages. And regardless of your beliefs, religion, gender, occupation, education, or any other things, it will help you to reach a state, where you can enjoy better health and greater happiness.

I envision that if a larger percentage of the people on the planet were healthier, the planet would be an even better place to live. You might ask how?

Simple! When you are healthier, you will think, act, and live more wisely. The decisions that you will take would be more prudent, efficient, effective, sustainable, and inclusive. Further, when you are happier, chances are you will also spread a little happiness around you. All of this will help you and also the other people in your neighbourhood, community, geography, and region to lead a better life.

Isn't that a win-win for all?

So, make note that when you are reading this book and working to improve your health, you are not just helping yourself; you are also making the world a better place - to live, work, and play.

Over the next few chapters, we will discuss the areas, which you need to work in order to bring the desired change in your health and fitness. This will help you to build and maintain good health as you grow older.

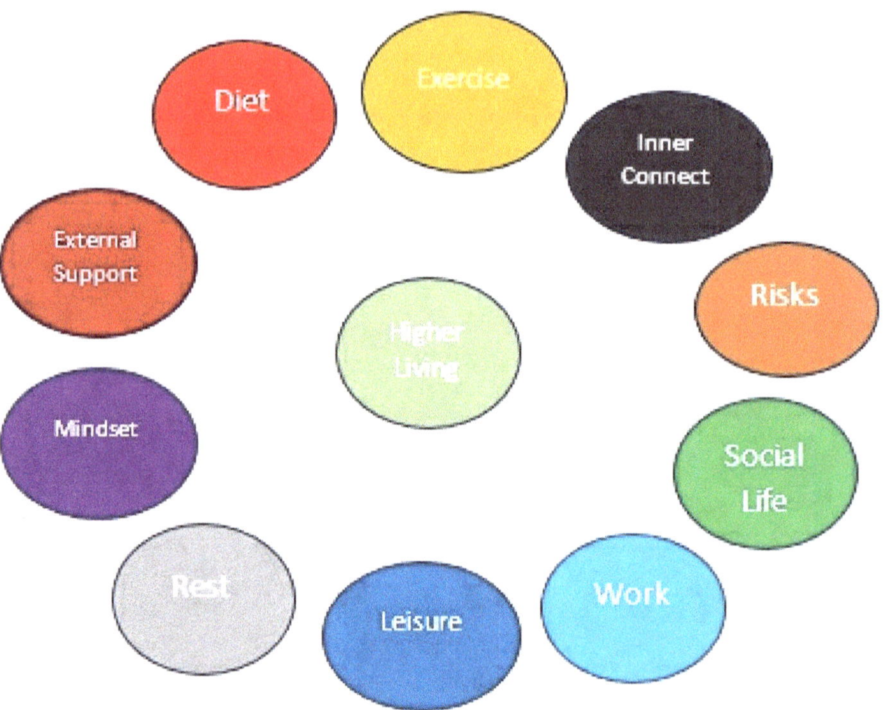

Diet
Exercise
Inner Connect
External Support
Higher Living
Risks
Mindset
Social Life
Rest
Leisure
Work

CONTENTS

PRACTICE HEALTHY EATING

"Eat your food as your medicine. Otherwise, you have to eat medicine as your food." — Steve Jobs

Watch What You Eat And Drink

Have you heard about terms like input and output? Some of you would have guessed what I am trying to say. For those who didn't, let me explain!

You provide petrol as an input to your car (I know world has now moved to gas and electricity to a large extent), and it gives you movement. Assume you mixed soda with petrol and fed your car. Now see how far you are able to drive. If you are lucky, you may be able to use the car normally for some time. But after some time, the ill effects will start showing up.

In the same manner, what you eat and drink is very important for your movement. When you are young, you may be able to get away with eating just about anything. But once you hit your 30's, you will realize the effects of junk eating. If you are lucky, you may be able to avoid any ill effects of unhealthy foods till you are in your 40s. But sooner or later, you will start to see how poor food choices can reduce your efficiency and quality of your life.

And what you eat not only affects your movement but all the areas of your life – health, wealth, relationships, performance, happiness, thought process, and more

On the other hand, if you eat the right food, then also you will see a change in your life. The only difference, here the changes would be positive.

Identify Junk Foods

Now, many of you may not know what exactly is junk and hence it is important to identify them in first place. Only when you know unhealthy foods, can you then avoid them. Below is a list of some of the unhealthiest food items that you might be consuming daily.

1. Refined wheat flour - Also referred to as all-purpose flour, refined wheat flour is deficient in micro and macronutrients. This deficiency can result in various health issues such as weight gain, elevated blood sugar levels, inflammation, cardiovascular problems, and digestive disorders. Furthermore, it contains a high amount of alloxan, a substance known to trigger diabetes. Consistent intake of refined flour can potentially lead to inflammation and the development of type-2 diabetes.

2. Sugar - Sugar is often referred to as an 'empty calorie' because it lacks vitamins and minerals. Consuming too much sugar can lead to increased inflammation and oxidative stress in the body, potentially causing harm to various organs and tissues.

3. Soft Drinks - Soft drinks, which typically contain high amounts of sugars, can contribute to various health issues such as weight gain, non-alcoholic fatty liver disease, and diabetes. Additionally, they are associated with a heightened risk of developing heart disease.

4. Packaged biscuits, wafers, and similar food stuff - These items frequently include harmful components such as refined flour and sugar. They are also typically rich in unhealthy fats and sodium, which can contribute to a variety of health problems, including heart disease, hypertension, and obesity.

The above list is not exhaustive as there are other items too that are not good for your health.

Understand The Nutrition Labels And Ingredients

At this point, I want to talk about packaged food items once again. I want to also let you know how you can identify what are the contents of a product and how to identify if it is unhealthy for you.

Pick up any packaged food item and look at its nutritional details and ingredients.

If you carefully scan the label, you can see the ingredients in the product. The components are listed in decreasing order of their percentage in the food item. In some cases, even the percentages of these ingredients are mentioned besides them.

Along with the ingredients, you will also be able to see the nutritional information of the food item. It provides the weights of various nutrients like carbohydrates, sugars, proteins, fat, and more in the food item.

Though there are lot of things you can see in the nutrition label and ingredients, you should be notice carefully for things like 'added sugars,' 'refined wheat flour,' and 'trans fats.' As their excessive intake can lead to health issues like obesity, heart disease, and diabetes. So, these are your unhealthy food items.

Now, once you know what food products are not good for your health, you can start to avoid it and increase the consumption of the items that are good for your health.

So, remember, understanding nutrition labels is the first step towards making healthier food choices. And, the next time you pick up a packaged food item, take a moment to read the label.

Find Alternative To Junk Foods

If it was so easy to eat healthy food than the whole world would be eating salads all day. But it is not that straight forward.

I agree that you cannot do away with sweets completely; you cannot totally avoid snacks and beverages also. But what if I told you there is a healthier alternative to the above items that gives you a similar effect. Then it would be easier for you to leave the junk food items and transition to a better alternative.

Here are some sample alternatives:

1. Whole Wheat Flour (for refined wheat flour).
2. Honey and Jaggery Powder (for sugar).
3. Lemonade (for soft drinks).
4. Home-made snacks like roasted chivda (for packaged snacks).

There are a lot more items that can be added to the list above. You just need to find them.

So, find and choose healthy.

Combine Health And Taste

There was a survey, which I read on the media. It said that even taste is important for your health. It found that if you eat food that does not satisfy your taste buds, you may not be able to maintain good health. I am not sure as to what extent this is true. But even if it is true, you still have options. There are food items that are both healthy and tasty.

Kanda Poha and Foxnuts are amazing examples in snacks. Dal Baati is another food item that meets both the criteria. To add more to the list, you have matar paneer and makki-ki-roti sarson-ka-saag. I have even seen puri(of paani puri) made of whole wheat at some places. I can keep adding, but I hope you get the point.

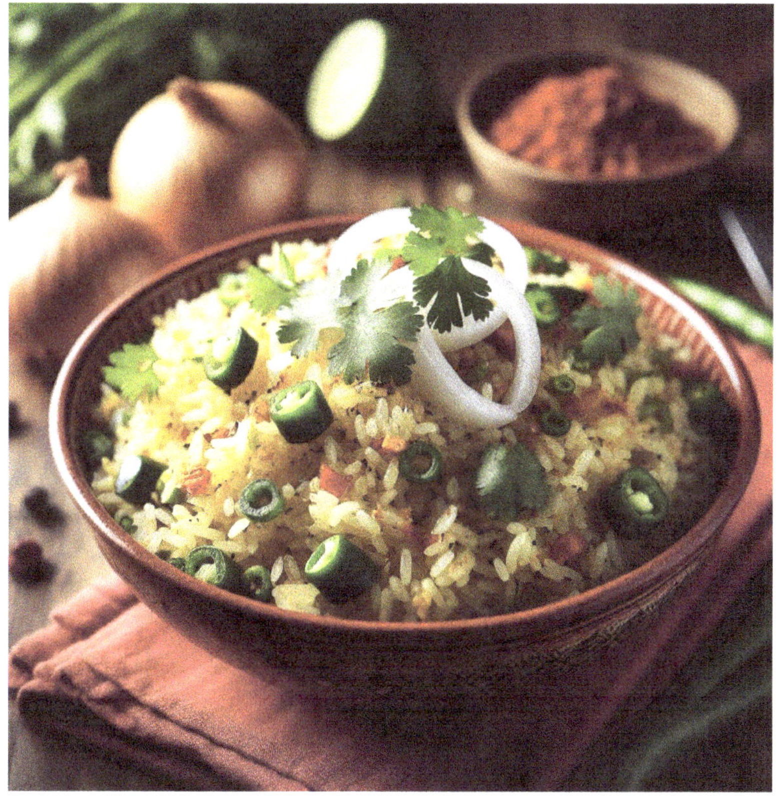

Kanda Poha

Kanda Poha, a beloved dish from Maharashtra in India, is made from 'Poha' or flattened rice, onions (known as 'Kanda' in Marathi), peanuts, green chillies, and various spices. The preparation involves washing the rice, caramelizing the onions, and then adding the damp rice to the pan, seasoning it with salt, sugar, coriander, and lemon juice. There are variations of this dish, such as Batata Poha (with potatoes) and Kanda Batata Poha (with onions and potatoes). This dish holds cultural significance in Maharashtra, being a staple

*breakfast and tea-time snack, and is often
served during arranged marriage meetings.*

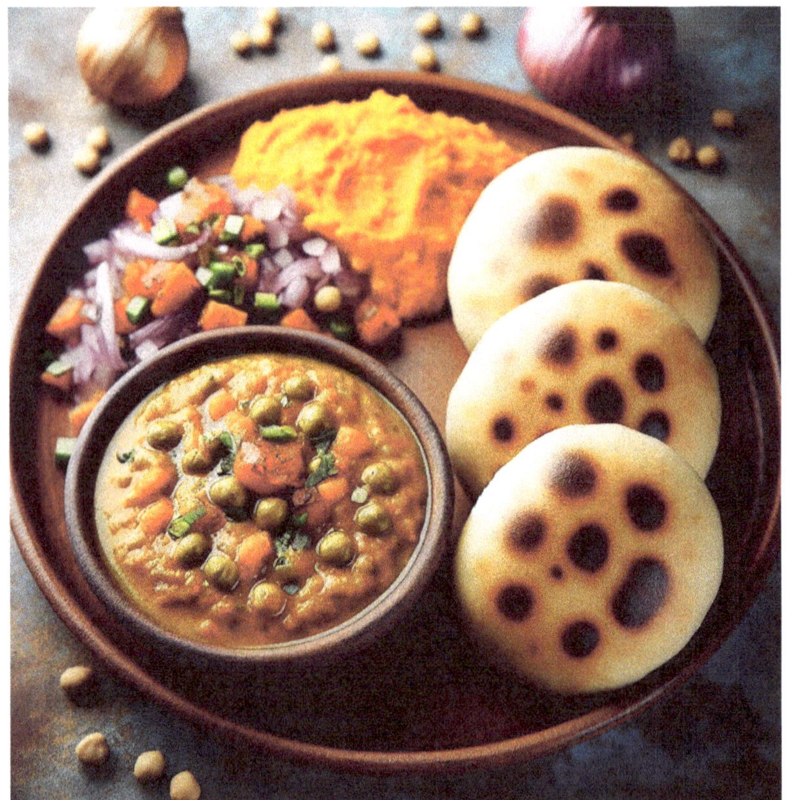

Dal Baati Chokha

*Dal Baati Chokha, a traditional dish from
the Indian subcontinent, is particularly
cherished in Rajasthan and Bihar. The dish
comprises three key elements: Baati, small
balls of wheat dough baked in a tandoor and
served with ghee; Dal, a spicy lentil curry
garnished with red chili tadka and garlic
chutney; and Chokha, a dish of mashed
potatoes seasoned with various spices. This*

*delightful combination offers a unique culinary
experience that has won the hearts of many.*

Most of the food items listed in the last two sections are Indian dishes. So, do not be disappointed if you cannot identify them. And you do not necessarily need to eat the same products. You can definitely try. But no compulsion! They are provided just as examples. Feel free to find healthy alternatives based on your own geographical and cultural settings.

Have A Balanced Diet

Avoiding unhealthy food and replacing it with healthier alternatives is definitely important. But then, it is also equally important to have a balanced diet.

You should continue to consume all types of vegetables, fruits, pulses, dal, nuts. Your water intake should be adequate. Basically, your body should receive all the vital nutrients that you need – proteins, carbs, fats, vitamins, minerals, and of course water.

And since no single food item may be able to provide everything that your body needs, a mix platter works great.

Additionally, in order for certain food items to show an impact on your body, you should even have it in requisite amount. Take for example, walnuts. You might be eating walnuts to get the benefits of omega-3 fatty acids from it. But if you consume too little, you may not notice the positive effect. Same goes for over eating. The key here is to try and find the right quantity. You can research, talk to your doctor, or even listen to your body to know the right amount to be consumed.

Have A Proper Eating Time

Should you eat a heavy food at dinner? Should you eat right before going to bed?

For those who are wondering about the answers to the above questions: 1. You should not eat heavy food at dinner 2. You should also leave a gap of 2-3 hrs between your dinner and bed time.

There are actually lot of things that you can work on the timing part of your food intake. I will leave it to you to find the best practices that works for you.

Aim to have breakfast between 6:00 to 9:45 a.m., and if needed, a snack around 10 to 11 a.m. Lunch is best around 1 p.m., and dinner should ideally be around 6 p.m. to 8 p.m., leaving a 2-3 hour gap before bedtime. Consistency in meal times and a 3-5 hour gap between meals can aid digestion and maintain blood sugar levels. Remember, these are guidelines and individual needs may vary.

DO REGULAR EXERCISE

"The pain you feel today will be the strength you feel tomorrow."
— Arnold Schwarzenegger

Exercise is like a medicine. And just like you brush your teeth and take a bath regularly, exercise also needs a regular inculcation in your life.

You need to start. And then slowly make it a habit. You can choose the exercises that suits you the best.

Walking

Start with 15-30 minute walks, 3-5 days a week. Gradually increase time or pace.

Walking is an exercise which is so simple that anyone can do it. All you need to do is wear a flip flop or a shoe, and get going. Do you think it is difficult?

In fact, even when you are feeling sleepy, you will still be able to complete a 40 minutes walking exercise without much effort.

On a lighter note, a lot of people actually do sleep walking.

Coming back to the point – walking is the easiest exercise in the world that anyone can do. And there are lot of benefits to it. Some of them are listed below.

- Increased cardiovascular fitness.
- Reduced body fat.
- Improved management of diabetes.
- Reduced stress levels.

Jogging

*Begin with alternating jogging and walking.
Increase jogging intervals over time.*

What you can achieve through walking, you may be able to get the same benefit from jogging in less than half the time. But make sure, you use a good shoe with enough cushion if you plan to jog. People with knee pains or joint problems should speak to their doctor before starting to jog.

If you are older than 40 or have any diseases, you should also consult your doctor before jogging.

Running

*Start with a run/walk method. Gradually
increase running intervals.*

This is even 1 step ahead than jogging. It can get your heart beat up in no time. But like jogging, this too is a little high impact on your joints. So, take your own call before practicing this.

Make sure to consult your doctor and also use the right shoe before you head for a run.

Older people need to be more careful before they decide to run. And should definitely consult their doctor before practicing running.

Stretching

Begin with basic stretches. Hold each stretch for about 30 seconds.

As a slow-paced controlled physical activity, stretching involves moving or holding parts of the body for the purpose of lengthening the muscles.

It improves flexibility and posture, and reduces muscle imbalances. It can alleviate body aches, back pain, and strengthen back muscles. Additionally, it provides stress relief by loosening tight muscles caused by stress.

If you plan to do go for a walk, jog, or a run, it would be wise to do a little warm up by stretching to prepare your body for the physical exercise.

Zumba

Familiarize yourself with Latin-based dances. Learn Zumba at home through DVDs or YouTube.

For those who need fun, Zumba is your go to exercise. It clubs dance and exercise together.

It is a popular and effective exercise that combines dance and aerobic movements.

Here are some of the key benefits of Zumba: Full-Body Workout, Calorie and Fat Burning, Builds Endurance, Improves Cardiovascular Fitness, Improved Blood Pressure, Boosts Mood, Tones Your Entire Body, and Improves Coordination and Dance Skills.

FIND THE INNER CONNECT

"The key to your deepest happiness is living a life in alignment with your true self." — Ralph Waldo Emerson

You are taught about the importance of networking by everyone. You try to make connections at work, at play, and in your communities. But sometimes, you lose connection with your own self. And this connection with your own self is ever more important that all the other connections put together.

Yoga

Start with a beginner's yoga class or video. Begin with basic poses, focusing on proper alignment and breathing. As your flexibility and strength improve, you can try more advanced poses.

A lot of people see yoga as just a set of poses. But there is more to it than what meets the eye. Yoga is a way of life. Besides that, for your fitness, it can bring very big transformations at all levels of your being.

Yoga is about being one with yourself. It works to strengthen your nervous system, exercise your internal glands, and can be an exercise for your whole body.

Meditation

Start with just a few minutes a day. Find a quiet, comfortable place, close your eyes, and focus on your breath. As your concentration improves, you can increase the duration.

In this world, where you are bombarded with thousands of events from hundreds of different sources, how do you find focus? The answer is meditation.

Mudra

Start by learning a few basic mudras, such as Gyan Mudra (for knowledge) or Prana Mudra (for energy). Practice each mudra for a few minutes a day, focusing on the sensations in your fingers and body.

Mudra is a little lesser-known methodology for fitness than Yoga and Pranayama. It basically works to directly balance the 5 different elements in your body - air, water, earth, space, and fire.

Pranayama

Start with simple breathing exercises, such as Anulom Vilom (alternate nostril breathing) or Kapalbhati (skull shining breath). Practice each exercise for a few minutes a day, focusing on your breath.

Breath or Pran is the central theme in pranayama. It also falls in the same group of exercise as Yoga, Meditation, and Mudra. If you can practice all of them, that can be really great.

Look Within

Start by setting aside a few minutes each day for self-reflection. This could be through journaling, meditation, or simply sitting quietly.

Most Human beings look outside. A very few ever try and look inside. I mean there is a whole world within you. And if you neglect this microcosm inside yourself, you may be missing out on a lot of things.

Listen To Your Body

Start by paying attention to how your body feels throughout the day. Notice any signs of stress, fatigue, or discomfort, and adjust your activities accordingly.

Your body always sends you signals for what it feels are good for you and what is not. It tells you when you need rest and when you need to work. All you need to do is to tune your frequency to hear what your body is saying. In simple terms, keep a look for signs that your body shows in the form of stress, fatigue, happiness, unhappiness, clarity, confusion, obesity, fitness, headache, insomnia, etc

And it will really work in your favour throughout your life.

ENGAGE IN WORK

"Whatever your life's work is, do it well. A man should do his job so well that the living, the dead, and the unborn could do it no better."   — Martin Luther King, Jr.

All work and no play make Jack a dull boy. But then, all play and no work will not necessarily give any different results, unless you are a professional sportsperson.

So, it is extremely important that you work.

Work For The Money

In order to pay bills and plan for the future, everyone needs money. Some are fortunate to have an abundance of it, but still, they also need to work to make more money. Because, growth is life. And if growth is not in question, then even to maintain your wealth, you need to do some work. Because if you are wealthy and you are not working then inflation will erode the actual value of your wealth without you even realising it.

Consider the story of Elon Musk, the CEO of SpaceX and Tesla. He is known for his immense wealth, but he didn't achieve his success by resting on his laurels. Despite having enough money to live comfortably for the rest of his life, Musk continues to work tirelessly on his ventures. His work ethic and continuous pursuit of growth serve as a testament to the idea that work is necessary for maintaining and increasing wealth.

Work For The Soul

Next is working for your soul. Not all work nourishes your soul. A majority of the people are not even lucky enough to be able to do a work that nourishes their soul.

There are lot of work that can nourish your soul. These can be any business, community work, charity, or volunteer work that is done primarily to enrich other peoples' lives or to make this world a better place. It can also be for anything else that falls in the category of good cause or the one that satisfies your soul.

Take the example of Mother Teresa. She dedicated her entire life to serving the poor and needy, a job that didn't earn her money, but nourished her soul. Her work made a significant difference in the lives of many and brought her immense personal satisfaction and peace.

Work At All Ages

A lot of people retire completely from work after a certain age. Though it is completely understandable to be practical and not engage in very demanding work as you age, it is not wise to become completely passive as you become old.

Agreed, that most of the people may not like to do a job or run a business after a certain age. But then, there are a lot of work – social, household, community, charity, mentoring – that can still be pursued even at very old ages.

This will keep your mind sharp and body fit even when you cross your 60s and 70s.

An example could be Harlan Sanders, better known as Colonel Sanders of KFC. He franchised his company, Kentucky Fried Chicken, at the age of 62. Despite the challenges, he continued to work well into his old age, proving that age is not a barrier to success or productivity.

BUILD A SOCIAL LIFE

"Shared joy is a double joy; shared sorrow is half a sorrow."
— Swedish Proverb

Spend Time With Family And Friends

You may become a Billionaire. However, if you do not have a person who you can call friend or family, your wealth may not have a lot of real meaning. So, make sure to find some time to spend it with your near and dear ones.

A lot of people think that they will first work to become wealthy and then they will have all the free time in the world to spend with their family and/or friends. I feel, most likely this may not work. Because, all relationships need time and nurturing, to build and also to maintain it. Additionally, you may not know where your family or friends will be when your right time comes.

If you have no family or friend, you can still adopt a pet and make him your friend. And you can do it even if you have a family or a friend. The two are not mutually exclusive.

Consider Bill Gates, co-founder of Microsoft. Despite being one of the richest people in the world, Gates has often spoken about the importance of his family and friends. He has been quoted saying that his relationships with his family and friends are his greatest source of happiness, not his wealth or business success.

Join A Community Or A Group

There is a different level of happiness and achievement, when you do something as a part of a team or a group. Though, some people prefer solitude compared to being in a group, it is still worthwhile to do some activities as a part of a group. Additionally, in the process, you may even end up building friendships and contacts that may benefit you for life.

Some of the things that are really suited to group work are travelling, eating, and social work. There may be many more. But hope this gives you an idea.

Oprah Winfrey is a renowned media executive, actress, talk show host, television producer, and philanthropist. She is best known for her talk show, "The Oprah Winfrey Show," which holds the record for being the highest-rated television program of its kind in history. Winfrey has consistently emphasized the importance of community, frequently using her influential platform to unite people. Her active leadership in community activities and groups has not only enriched her own life but has also made a positive impact on the lives of countless others.

FIND TIME FOR LEISURE

"The end of labour is to gain leisure." — Aristotle

Sports

Sports are yet another way to maintain general fitness at all ages. There are plenty of them, some indoor and others are outdoor sports.

Swimming, Badminton, Basketball, Table Tennis, Tennis, Golf, and Chess are some great examples in sports.

Below are some of the most popular sports in the world and their benefits.

Sport	Physical Health Advantages	Mental Health Advantages
Golf	Enhances heart health, supports weight loss, increases flexibility, and improves balance.	Boosts mental well-being by alleviating stress, enhancing mood, and promoting social interactions.
Swimming	Decreases the risk of overall mortality by 24% and improves body composition and blood lipids.	Boosts mood, alleviates stress, and enhances self-esteem.
Tennis	Enhances aerobic capacity, supports weight loss, improves balance, and enhances motor control.	Boosts mood, alleviates stress, and enhances self-esteem.

Table Tennis	Enhances balance, agility, and coordination, and strengthens muscles in the arms, legs, and core.	Enhances mental well-being by reducing stress, boosting mood, and fostering social connections.
Cricket	Enhances strength, improves endurance, and improves balance and coordination.	Enhances teamwork skills and reduces stress.
Badminton	Enhances aerobic fitness, improves muscle tone and strength, and increases speed and agility.	Boosts mood, alleviates stress, and enhances self-esteem.
Football	Positively impacts body composition, blood lipids, fasting blood glucose, blood pressure, resting cardiovascular function, cardiorespiratory fitness, and bone strength.	Promotes teamwork skills and alleviates stress.
Basketball	Enhances muscular endurance, builds healthy bones, improves balance and coordination.	Enhances teamwork skills and reduces stress.

Please remember that the benefits can vary depending on the intensity and frequency of the sport. And always consult with a healthcare professional before starting any new sport or fitness regimen, in case you have any concerns.

Hobbies

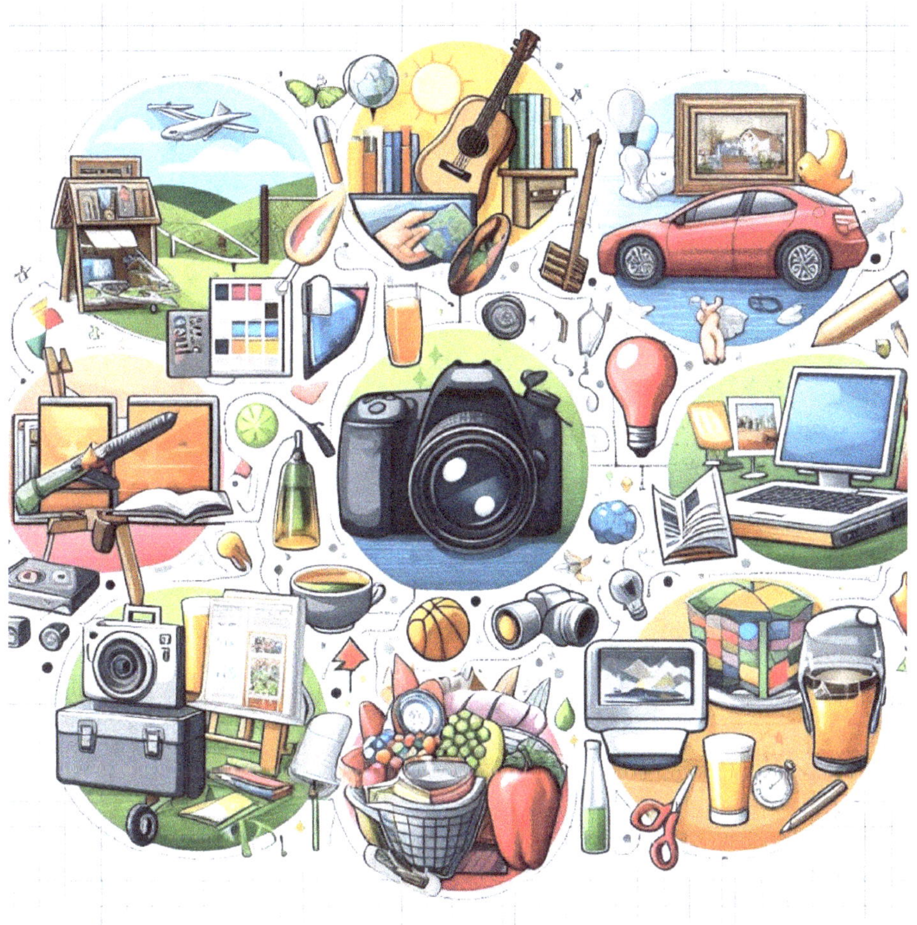

I am sure you must have read the saying 'All work and no play makes jack a dull boy'. And it is not incorrect to say so. Personally, I cannot imagine only working all my life and not engaging in any leisure activities. Life would be so boring if that was the case. You yourself will hate to live like that. So, why not engage in some amazing hobbies?

Others need not dictate to you, which hobbies to indulge in. It is completely your choice. And it can be anything from gardening to coin collecting to bird watching and so many more things. Just find your calling and take the plunge.

Travel And Vacation

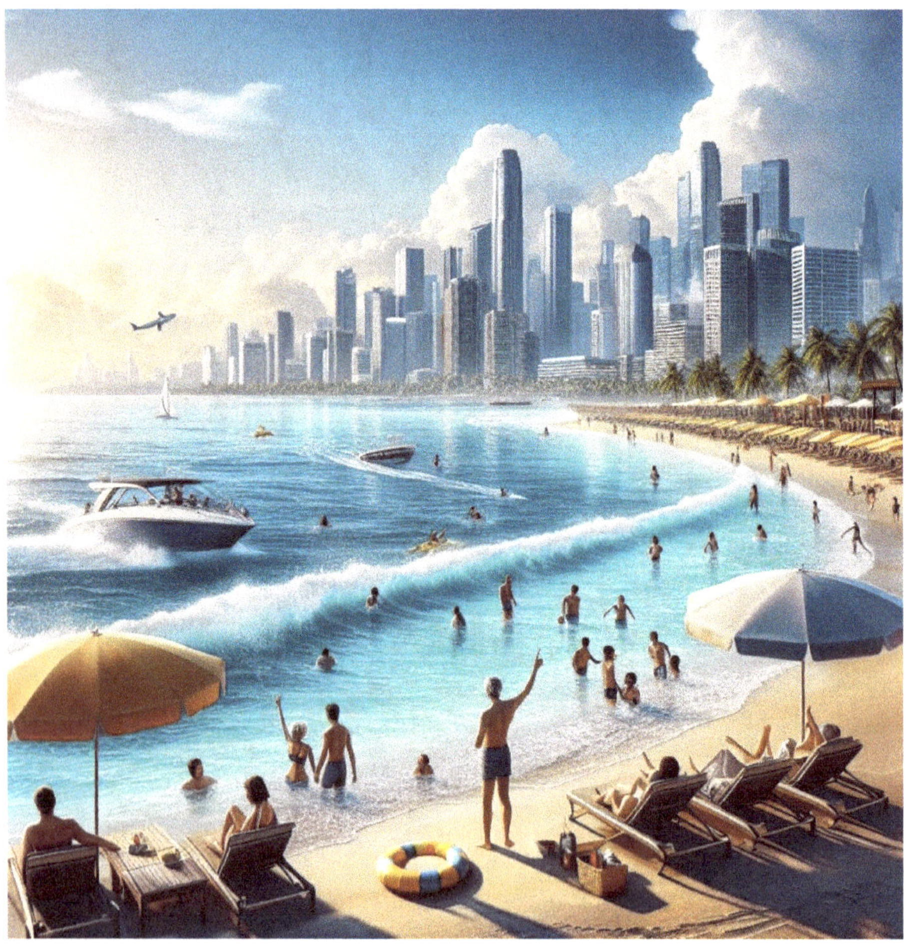

We have to accept the fact that life does get boring sometimes when we are surrounded by the same people and environment every day. So, Travel and Vacations becomes important here. It gives you a change from the mundane and adds a punch of zest to your life. Breathtaking views of mountains, lakes, oceans are sure to fill your heart and soul with a flavour of joy and happiness. So, make time for it. If not very far, then at least you can visit the other end of your town or city, once in a while.

TAKE ADEQUATE REST

"Wisdom is knowing when to have rest, when to have activity, and how much of each to have."
— Sri Sri Ravi Shankar

Proper Rest And Sleep

Life is full of struggles. Everyone is fighting some or the other war - big or small - everywhere. All of this takes a toll on you physically and mentally. In order for you to again replenish yourself to be able to take on the next day, you need rest. Sleep is when a lot of the automatic processes in your body runs in the background to service your body.

An important point to note here is that either a lack or excess of sleep may not be in the best for your health.

Though everyone has their own preferences regards to the sleep timings, if you were to ask me, I will suggest going early to bed and rising up early.

Even the duration of the sleep should be balanced – not too little and not too much. Based on individual's age, work, and other factors, 6 to 8 hrs sleep is recommended for most. For very old people, it may be difficult to sleep more but you should still make it a point to sleep at least 5-6 hrs.

Prioritize Yourself

Everyone in this world is chasing their own dream. Your boss, friend, wife, co-worker, and others have their own plans or vision for life. And each of them would somehow also try to drive things as per their vision and plans. Though it is completely fine to make small accommodations to have things moving ahead, it should not be at the price of deprioritizing yourself. So, prioritize yourself. Because if you won't, then no one else will.

Start declining(politely) invitations to events and parties that does not serve your interest. Same for a lot of other things that are constantly asking for your time.

HAVE A GREAT MINDSET

"It's a funny thing about life, once you begin to take note of the things you are grateful for, you begin to lose sight of the things that you lack." — Germany Kent

Be Positive

It sounds really simple. But the fact is, it is not that easy for people to stay positive always. We live in a world surrounded by other people, environments, events and so on. However, with practice and effort, you can become a more positive person. Slowly, you can also become positive in all situations and circumstances. And this can change you, your body, your mind, and your life.

So, be positive always.

Here, you can also try and use Ksepana Mudra, if you want to. It can assist you in becoming more positive.

> *"Positive thinking is a valuable tool that can help you overcome obstacles, deal with pain, and reach new goals." — Amy Morin*

Have A Little Fun

After working in the corporate world for over a decade, I forgot having fun. It was only when I got to work in startup that I was re-introduced to fun. Having fun does not necessarily means going out and partying. To me, it simply meant enjoying whatever I am doing and being young at heart.

> *"Just play. Have fun. Enjoy the game." — Michael Jordan*

Laugh

It is said that 'Laughter is the Best medicine'. It is actually true. There was a time when I use to think that laughing does not look sober. So, I used to laugh less. But I have now found that, it is completely fine to laugh when you get a chance to do so. It is just you being yourself.

If you find it hard to life, there are plenty of people around the world who are trying to make it easy for you.

> *"Laughing is good exercise. It's like jogging on the inside."* — *Kurt Vonnegut*

Cry

Just like laughing, crying is also an expression. So, if you feel like crying, go and cry. If you are not comfortable doing so in presence of other people, you can cry someplace alone.

> *"Tears are the summer showers to the soul."* — *Alfred Austin*

Be Active

Life is very short. You may not even complete a century. And you should really try and accomplish something in your lifespan. So, keep moving. There can be situations in life that can slow you down or decrease your motivation. But you should really make it a point to be active always.

> *"Being active every day makes it easier to hear that inner voice."* — *Haruki Murakami*

Be Like A River And Go With The Flow

I am always fascinated by rivers. How they keep on flowing in all weathers and terrains, is specially amazing to see. There are so many obstacles that comes in its path, but it just keeps flowing.

If you can make your life like a river, your life can also be better than the version you might be living today. On the other side, if you are not very active, chances are you may be susceptible to a lot of disease in this modern world. So, why not flow like a river and nourish the lives of those that you encounter during the journey? I say, there is absolutely nothing like it!

> *"I had no plans of any destination. I wish to flow like a river." — Lailah Gifty Akita*

Be A Giver

The world is trained to become a consumer - you get candies as a kid, educational institutions give you knowledge, banks give you loans, tv gives you entertainment and news, companies give you salaries, and so on. As you age, you keep becoming even bigger consumers. There is no limit to it.

Your life can be different if you start to think of becoming a producer.

Have you tried doing research on something and sharing that research knowledge with someone? Have you anytime thought of creating a product which can help other people? Have you tried to make someone else happy? Have you donated a meal to a needy? You do not need to be rich or highly successful to do that. You can do all of this at your scale. With this you become a producer, and that's where the magic starts. You will then start to experience the joy of giving.

So, go ahead and see how can you serve others.

> *"We make a living by what we get, but we make a life by what we give." — Winston Churchill*

Get The Driver Seat

Most of the people in this world have no plans of their own. And they just keep becoming part of someone else's plan. There is nothing wrong with this, if this approach is evident in a small part of your life. You can definitely join a company as an employee, get paid, and contribute to a company's mission. You can also accompany a friend on his trip to Hawaii or Miami. But this pattern should not be the significant hallmark of your life as a whole.

Do not let other people drive the significant decisions of your life. Everyone in this world looks for their interest and will possibly ignore any of your losses or disadvantages in the process. So, it becomes imperative that you safeguard your interests.

Having said that, you can still listen to other people's ideas, plans, dreams, and so on. However, you should be the one making the major decisions of your life.

*"You want to be in the driver's seat of
your own life because if you are not, life
will drive you." — Oprah Winfrey*

Choose Happiness Over Pleasure

There is a difference between happiness and pleasure.

Pleasure is when you felt good after buying a luxury car. Happiness is when your work improved the life of millions of people.

Sitting on a beach side with your friends and enjoying the nice breeze is happiness. Winning a lottery is not really happiness.

You can find happiness in the smallest of things in this world. You do not need to be a billionaire for that. But you definitely need a mindset to identify and experience that happiness.

And just to be clear, I agree that different people find happiness in different things. What I am trying to say is, you should identify the distinction between happiness and pleasure; and prioritize happiness.

By the way, you can still dream of buying a yacht or a jet. There is nothing wrong with that. But do not miss out on the happiness along the way to your dreams. And do not wait to become rich in order to feel happy.

Another important point to note here is: when you are healthy, you are implicitly happy. So, be healthy and you will increase the happiness index of your life.

Happiness is different from pleasure.
Happiness has something to do
with struggling and enduring and
accomplishing. — George A. Sheehan

Don't Stop Dreaming

When you were small, I bet you would have definitely dreamed of making it big and also achieving unbelievable feats. But as time passed, those dreams were killed. Either you killed it yourself or the world contributed in killing it.

Irrespective of what caused your dreams to vanish in thin air, you can still dream.

We all have heard of popular names like Elon Musk and Bill Gates.

You also know famous stars like Christiano Ronaldo, Lionel Messi, Jennifer Lopez, Selena Gomez, Taylor swift, Justin Bieber, and J.K Rowling.

All these people made it big because they kept their dreams alive in face of all adversities and all the problems they encountered year after year.

So, there is no reason why you should stop believing in our dreams. And if your dreams no longer exist, it is time to bring it alive.

> *"Never stop dreaming. Never stop listening to the music that is inside of you."* — *Debasish Mridha*

LIVE A HIGHER LIFE

"Simplicity of living plus high thinking leads to the greatest happiness." — Paramhansa Yogananda

Find A Purpose

Have you come across a few people who are very driven in whatever they are doing? And then there are others who just seems to be dragging themselves in order to accomplish even the smallest of work.

Find your purpose and then you can also become a highly driven person. There are good chances that you may even start to feel a lot more energetic in your life and work.

For some people their purpose can be to make their child a doctor, while for some others it can be to live a balanced life.

The list is endless. It's only you who can find your purpose; no other person can find it for you.

Associate With A Social Cause

It is true that everyone cannot lead and everyone cannot start a movement. So, what? Everyone does not need no either. There are already tons of readymade entities doing good work in a lot of areas to make this world a better place and to improve the lives of people. All you have to do is join the movement. Isn't that easy?

And you need not necessarily put time; you can also contribute by way of financial assistance or material assistance. In fact, the assistance and association can take many different forms.

Imbibe Values

If you live a life that is devoid of basic human values, then you surely are not living a great life. The worst part is, it will show up in your health.

It is like your body also reacts to things that are no aligned with basic principles of human life. For example, you can rob a person of his wealth and become a millionaire via illegitimate means or cheating. But deep within, you will know that you did not use the right means to become rich. This surely can reflect negatively on your health.

Some of the values which I can suggest you to make part of your life are: integrity, respect, honesty, kindness, gratitude, forgiveness, authenticity, compassion, empathy, equality, courage.

LEVERAGE EXTERNAL SUPPORT

"Do not suffer in silence. Somebody somewhere is willing and prepared to help in any way to encourage, empower, and support you." — Germany Kent

Get A Medical Assistance Where Required

There are a lot of things which you can solve. Perhaps if you had time to learn everything, you may not need a specialized person for any of your problems. But since your time in only limited and you cannot learn everything in-depth, for situations or problems where you are not able to make any progress for a long period of time, you can consider some medical assistance.

Speak To Someone You Trust

It is said that happiness increases and pain reduces, when shared. So, you can consider sharing some of your issues with the people you trust. This can help you in two ways: you may feel somewhat relieved and the person may also be able to provide some solutions that you could not find yourself.

God Is Always There

I know there are people who believe in God and those who don't. Additionally, there is also a set of people who neither believes nor disbelieves in God. And everyone has a right to believe in their beliefs.

For those, who believe in God. This part is for you.

There are times when things are really very difficult. All you see is darkness. And there is hardly anyone to help.

Here, when you seem to have exhausted all sources of external help, the almighty still exists for you. So, go and pray to him for support and kindness in those trying circumstances. And you surely should see some light ahead at the end of the tunnel.

For those, who are not sure or do not believe in the existence of God, you too can focus on the forces of the world that you believe in. And it can help you sustain the difficult situations in a similar way.

MANAGE RISKS

"The key to risk management is never putting yourself in a position where you cannot live to fight another day."

— Richard S. Fuld, Jr.

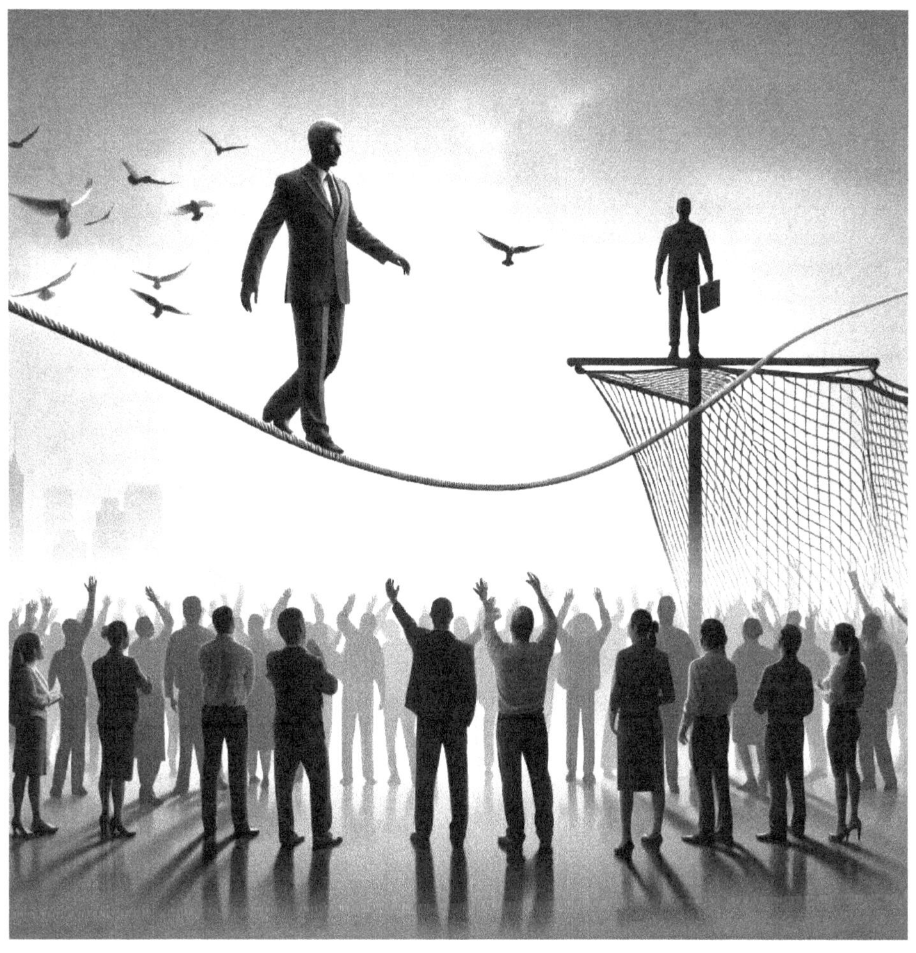

If you were to think of your life as a project, then your life will have some risks too.

Risk, in simple terms is anything that is uncertain. And while you cannot manage all the risks in life, there are some, which you can definitely manage.

The risk that I want to specifically talk about are events like loss of life and medical emergencies.

The first risk, if materializes can leave your family in a difficult financial situation, if you do not have a life insurance. This is especially significant if you are the sole bread winner in your family.

The second risk can wipe out all your earnings; and it can also leave you and your family stranded for money. This should not come as a surprise to you because everyone knows how large medical bills can grow in today's time.

Consider Opting For Basic Insurance

So, in order to lessen your worries, it is highly recommended that you make use of the tools like life insurance and health insurance. You do not need to opt for the most expensive coverages. But at the very least, a basic level of cover is recommended for all.

Though the above insurances will not improve your health directly, it will surely give you some peace, which will indirectly aid in your health.

Undergo Routine Health Tests

They say 'prevention is cure' and the saying is a cliché now. But that does not reduce its importance. Still, most of us really don't adhere to it.

A Lot of people fail to do something about their illnesses and diseases when they are at a nascent stage. And then they pay a hefty price for it later on.

Of course, I do not recommend going out and doing tests 365 days a year. And I am also not asking you to undergo tests the day right after you experience some issues. But, for any discomfort or signs provided by your body, you should undergo tests and visit a registered practitioner after few days or a month (depending on the issue) to catch the issues when they are young; and not when they become nasty.

Once the issue becomes chronic it will take a lot more of your time, effort, and money to cure the problem. It will be difficult too.

Try To Prevent Old Age Related Diseases

There are some diseases whose chances of occurrence increases as people age. Though there is no hard and fast rule. And there is no fixed set of diseases in this group. But based on some studies and research, some of the disease definitely pose a higher risk. And as such, you should try to prevent its occurrence.

Heart attacks, Dementia, Diabetes, Eye diseases, Kidney stones, Skin Diseases, and Bones & Joint Issues, are some of the diseases that are more prominent is people with higher age. But if you follow the guidelines provided in this book you should be in a good position to prevent their occurrence. Or worst, you would at least be able to decrease its severity or treat it in its early stages.

This is where your diet, exercise, regular health checkups, and discipline comes to your help. So, maintain and build good habits, so that you avoid the typical age-related diseases.

END NOTE

As we come to the end of the book, I want to share one more thing. And that is about the importance of making an effort.

A lot of people in the world suffer from bad health mostly because they do not put efforts. Look, the only direction you will go, if you do not consciously put effort to improve your health, is towards diseases and ill-health.

Sitting on the sofa and watching TV is easier. And for good things, you need to make efforts.

So, with all the knowledge shared in this book, it is your job to make the necessary efforts in the direction of health. Sure, it may not be easy. But it is definitely worth it.

Wishing you good health and happiness!

FAQS

1. Why is jaggery considered healthier than sugar?

Ans Jaggery is considered healthier than sugar for several reasons. They are listed below.

Nutrient Content: Jaggery, being an unrefined sugar, retains more minerals like iron, calcium, potassium, magnesium, manganese, zinc, and selenium from sugarcane juice. Sugar, on the other hand, loses these nutrients during its refining process.

Digestion: Jaggery is a complex sugar that is digested slowly, preventing a rapid spike in blood sugar levels. In contrast, sugar is absorbed instantly, leading to sudden blood sugar spikes.

Iron Source: Jaggery is a good source of plant-based iron, which is important for muscular function and energy boost.

Weight Management: Jaggery can boost metabolism and help burn fat, while sugar can lead to weight gain due to sudden blood sugar spikes.

Immunity Boost: Jaggery is rich in antioxidants that aid in building immunity and reducing the risk of diseases like cancer and dementia. It also helps reduce signs of aging. Sugar, however, provides empty calories with no nutritional value.

Cold and Infection Treatment: Jaggery's cleansing and anti-allergic properties can help treat cold, cough, and asthma by eliminating toxins and mucus from the lungs and respiratory tract. Sugar does not have these properties.

Please note that while jaggery has these benefits, it is still a form of sugar and should be consumed in moderation. Always consult with a healthcare professional or a dietitian for personalized advice.

2. I am nearing 50 now. Can I play sports?

Ans. Age should not be a constraint, unless you have any problems/illness that stops you from playing a sport. You can play friendly games or engage in low intensity sports. Swimming is a good example.

3. I cheated someone to become rich. What should I do?

Ans. In the first place, you should not have taken this route. But now that you have already cheated someone and became rich, you can try and return the wealth (principal and interest) to the person. How and how much? That is something you will need to figure.

Also, since you have now identified your negative actions, you should make amends for it. And forgive yourself. Also, make sure to choose better paths for your future goals.

4. How long should I wait before I take an external medical assistance for a health problem or goal?

Ans. It all depends on you and the problem. If you are having fever, you can see for a couple of days; if you have a little bit of acne on your face, you can see for a few weeks; if you collapsed while climbing stairs, you should go immediately; if you put on additional 1 kg weight in body in 1 year, you can track your weight changes for another year before visiting a doctor.

These are just some ideas and examples. You are the best person to decide, when to seek external support based on the problem and its severity.

5. Apart from the above, what else can I do for my overall health and fitness?

Ans. You can try to spend more time with the nature. Take for example, sunlight. Soaking in warm sunlight of the dawn and dusk can aid your health tremendously.

Besides sunbathing, visiting a green forest, camping on the river side, trekking on mountains, and enjoying sea side breeze can also be very refreshing and rejuvenating for your whole being.

6. Can you provide an example of associating with a social cause?

Ans. You can work as a teaching volunteer in a school of less privileged kids. You can spend time with people in an old age home. You can donate money to a relief fund. There are plenty.

7. I am not very rich. How can I donate for a cause?

Ans. You don't need to be a millionaire to donate. If you have 100 dollars, can you not give 1 dollar to a person in need. You just need a big heart to donate.

Note: I am not asking you to donate all your wealth. But to donate a proportionate amount based on your wealth.

8. I am a woman and I don't not find enough time for exercise after all the daily chores?

Ans. We all have 24 hrs in a day. No one has less or more. It all boils down to your priorities. If you think health is one of your priorities then you should make time for it.

9. Which is the best exercise according to you?

Ans. It is your personal choice. However, in my opinion, it is best to mix various forms of activities – sports, gym, yoga, stretching, running, and so on. It keeps you motivated and engaged. Because if you do the same exercise or activity daily for weeks and months, there are good chances you will get bored.

10. I drink a lot. Should I stop drinking completely?

Ans. Anything in excess can have ill effects on your health. And excess of alcohol is definitely something you should avoid.

It would be best for you to gradually reduce your alcohol intake and keep it to minimum.

11. I am suffering for bad health since a lot of years. Can I improve my health?

Ans. Why not? If you make efforts in the right direction, you should definitely be able to improve our health.

The improvement may not be drastic and might take time. But you should definitely see the results.

12. I want to wake up early. But I cannot even if I put an alarm?

Ans. The fact is: it is very difficult to wake up early if you sleep late. So, make it a point to sleep early and gradually your body clock will adjust to the new timings.

13. I have not been having enough water daily? How can I have enough water daily?

Ans. 3-4 litres of water daily is recommended for most of the people. You can keep multiple 1litre bottles and use it to track your daily consumption of water.

14. Can screen usage impact my health?

Ans. Yes, excessive screen times can have bad effects on your health. Take frequent breaks, and avoid night time screen usage. Try to spend more time of your day away from the screens.

15. I am 65 now. Is there a point improving my health now?

Ans. You can ask yourself why do you have to live with bad health. An age of 65 does not mean your life has come to an end.

If you keep fit at this age, you will live a better life for the remainder of your life. Else, you may not know how long you will live and will continue to suffer due to lack of health.

16. Are the suggestions and tips in this book targeted for any particular age group?

Ans. No, the details provided in this book can be used by all age groups. They are general suggestions and people should customize it as per their own needs.

Irrespective of your age, the information in this book should help you to age with good health.

17. There so many areas provided to work for good health? Can I not just go to gym and build health?

Ans. You may be able to build physical strength, which too may not last very long after you stop visiting the gym. So, it will most likely be insufficient to help you build complete fitness.

Also, your overall health encompasses your physical, mental, emotional, financial, social, and spiritual health.

So, working in a balanced way across all areas of your life will help you to achieve wholistic health and you will be able to have a much richer experience of life.

18. Can you recommend a good website on health and fitness?

Ans. There are plenty. I find Healthline to be a great source of information on health-related things.

19. I find it difficult to eat a lot of food items to consume a balanced diet. What can I do?

Ans. Though there should not be an excuse for not eating a balanced diet, there are certain food products you can consume to compensate for the same. Superfoods like Egg can come in handy at such times. They are packed with several important nutrients all in the same product.

20. I do not have a lot of money? Can I still age healthily?

Ans. You do not need to be a millionaire to stay healthy. As long as you are able to meet your basic needs and have some financial cushion, you can age healthily.

27. Are there any ways to feel relaxed when feeling stressed or uneasy?

Ans. You can also try to activate your vagus nerve   which can lead you to a state of feeling more relaxed and calm.

In order to do that, sit on a chair with a straight back, and hands on your thighs.

Breathe in deeply for 6 counts, then hold the breath for a count of 4. Next breathe out for a count of 8 and then hold that position for 6 counts.

Repeat the cycle for 5-10 minutes and you should experience calmness and relaxation.

You can also do this exercise in Sukhasana pose.

THANK YOU!

Hope this book will help you positively in your journey towards health and wellness in life.

If you enjoyed this book, do share it with your friends, family, and colleagues. It's a great way to spread knowledge and inspire others.

You may also add a review about the things that you liked in this book.

Other Books By Shiv Kumar

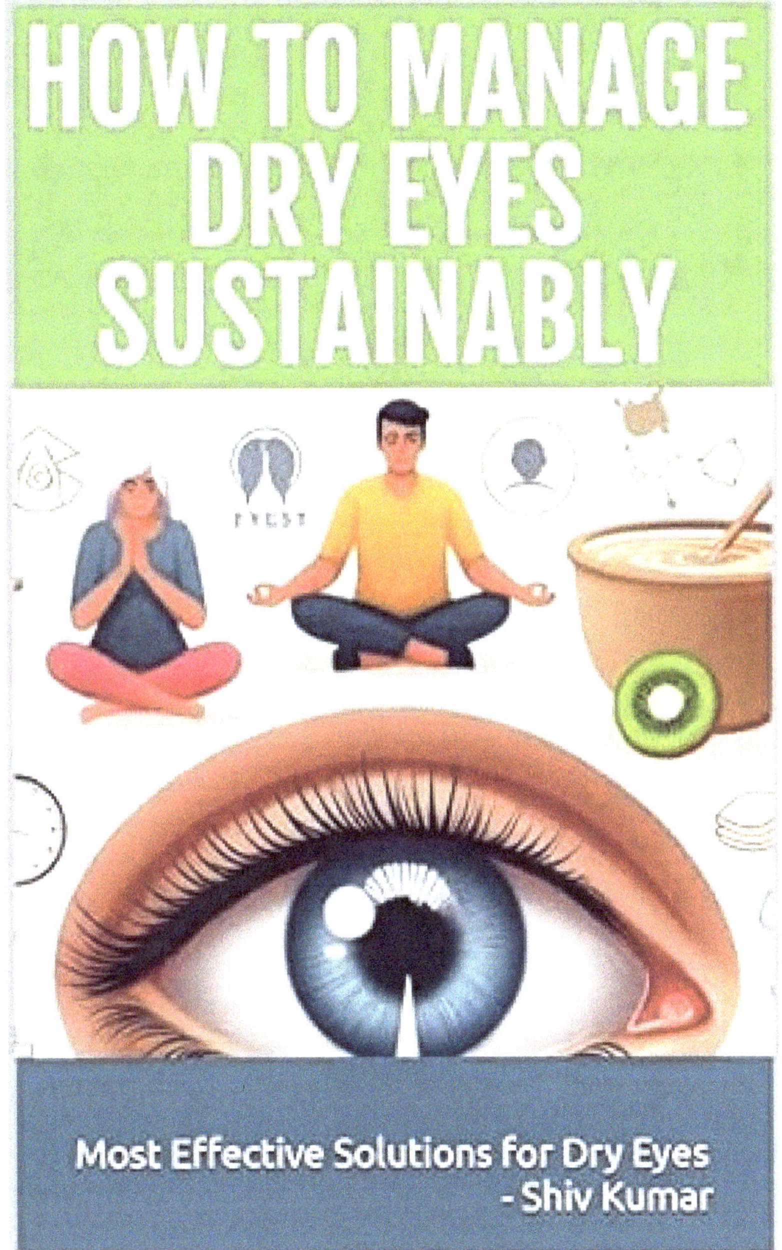

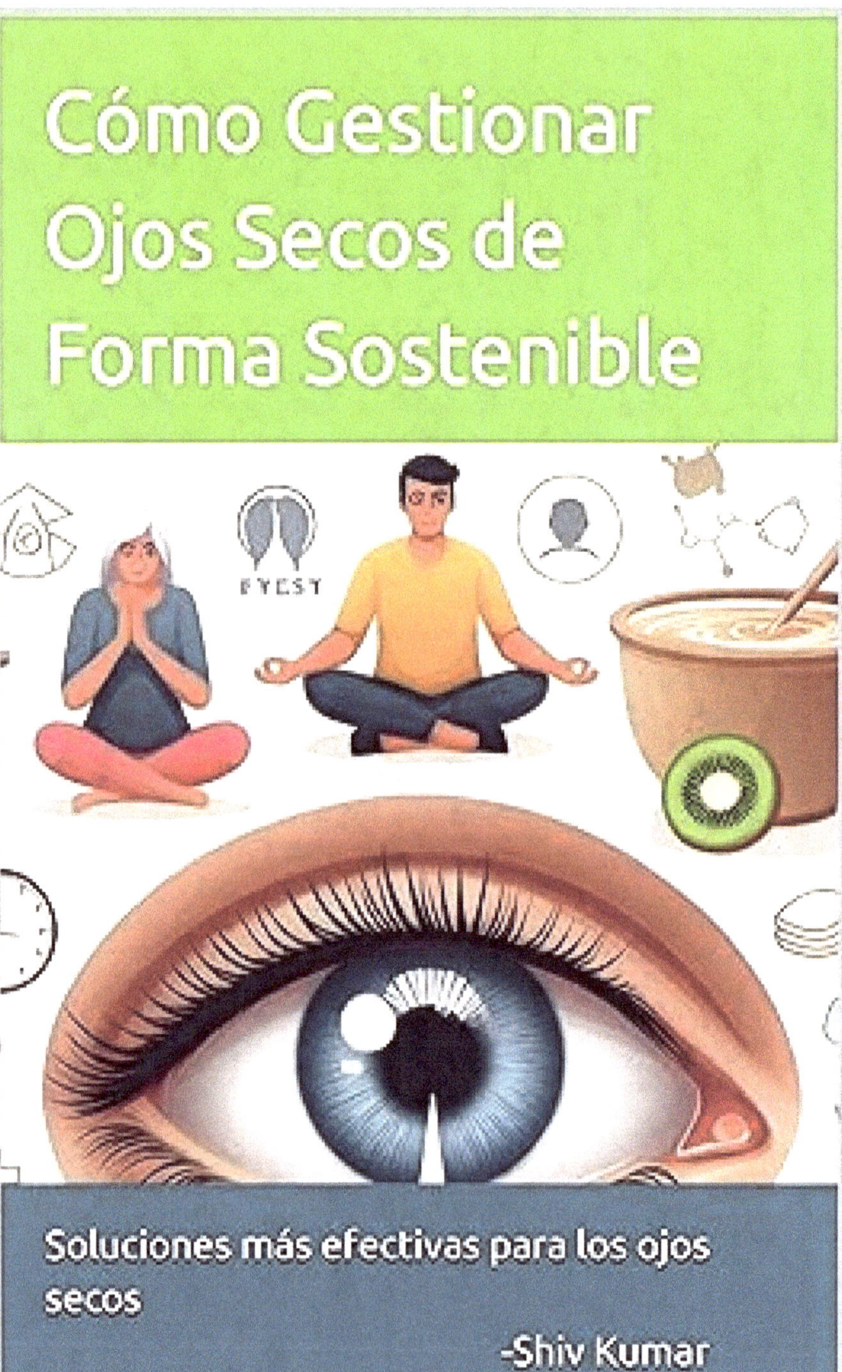

Cómo Gestionar Ojos Secos de Forma Sostenible
EYEST
Soluciones más efectivas para los ojos secos
-Shiv Kumar

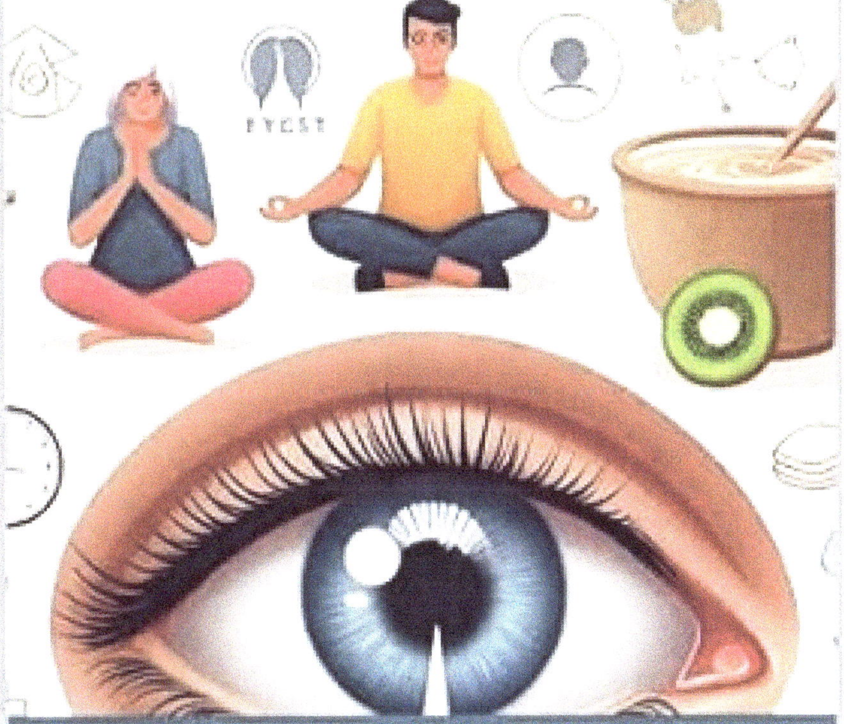
Wie verwaltet man Nachhaltig trockene Augen
Die wirksamsten Lösungen für trockene Augen
- Shiv Kumar

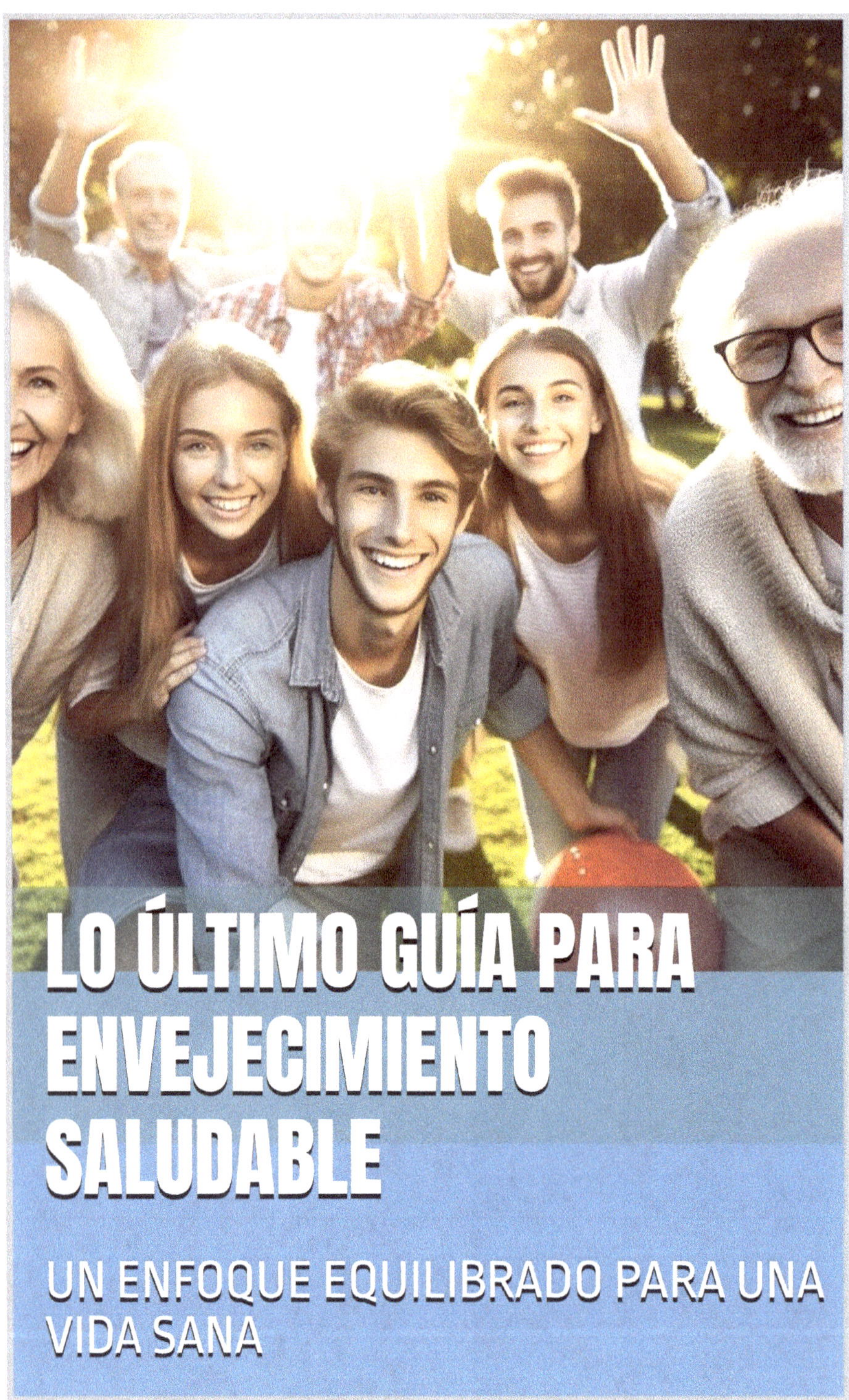

LO ÚLTIMO GUÍA PARA ENVEJECIMIENTO SALUDABLE
UN ENFOQUE EQUILIBRADO PARA UNA VIDA SANA

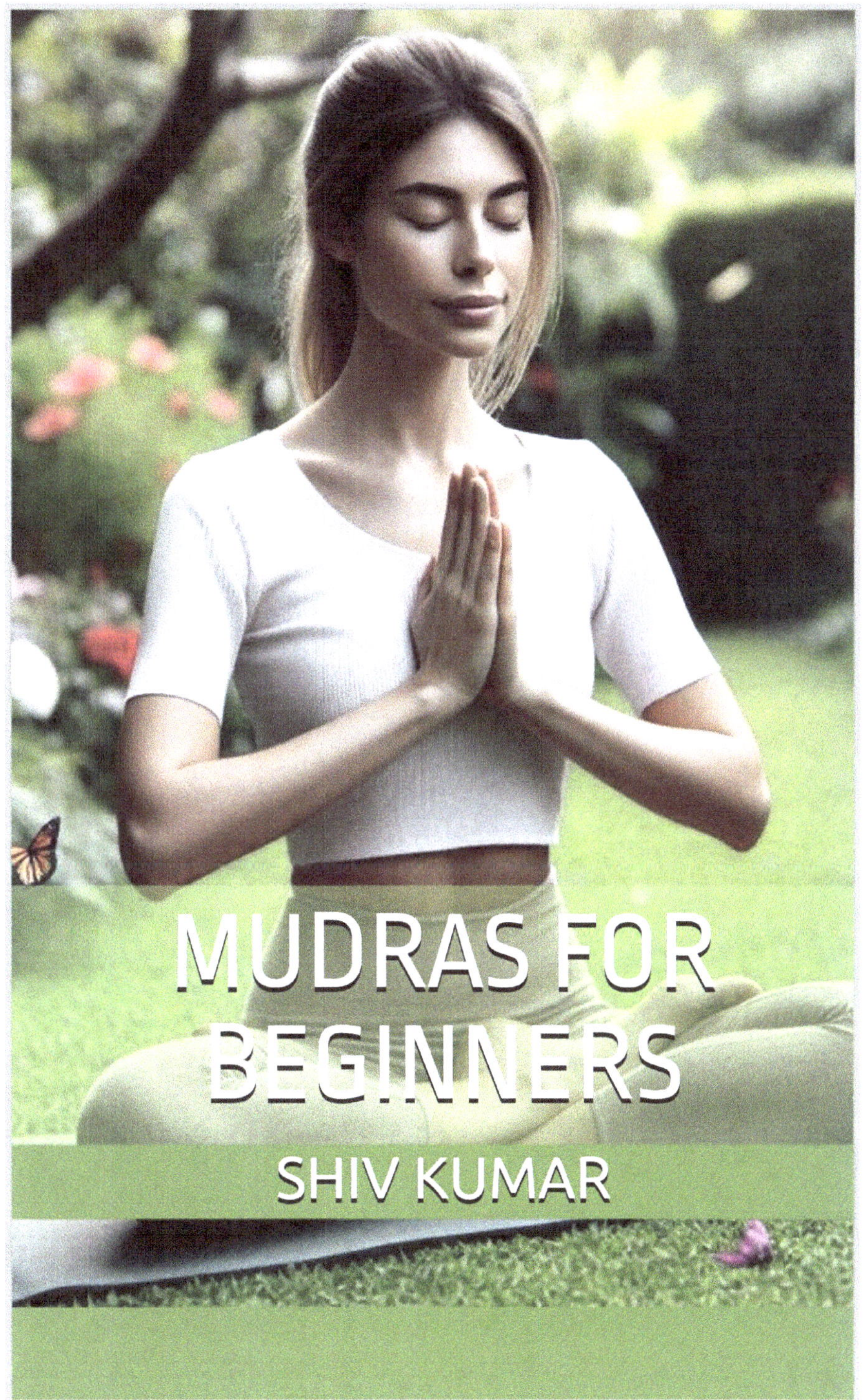
MUDRAS FOR BEGINNERS
SHIV KUMAR